HOME WORKOUTS FOR WOMEN

EXERCISES FOR TRAINING

FULL BODY

IN PICTURES

(1,2,3 parts)

INTRODUCTION

This booklet was designed for girls and women who can be engaged in a gym or any other exercise for physical activity. With our photo book you can make your body better. The book has exercises for full body and buttocks.

Each of these exercises you can perform at home, or in any other place. You will not need global props for this workout. And if you have children, you can work with them and this will be the additional load for you.

We offer to perform these exercises every in one day. Do not do all the exercises in a row, choose the ones that are comfortable for you and we showed you different variations of similar exercises so that each reader chooses the best for himself.

We suggest doing 3 rounds of 5-7 exercises 20 times each. Rest between rounds 3-5 minutes.

Do not rest between exercises for more than 20 seconds.

WE WILL BE FAMILIAR – JULIA.

YOUR PERSONAL TRAINER!

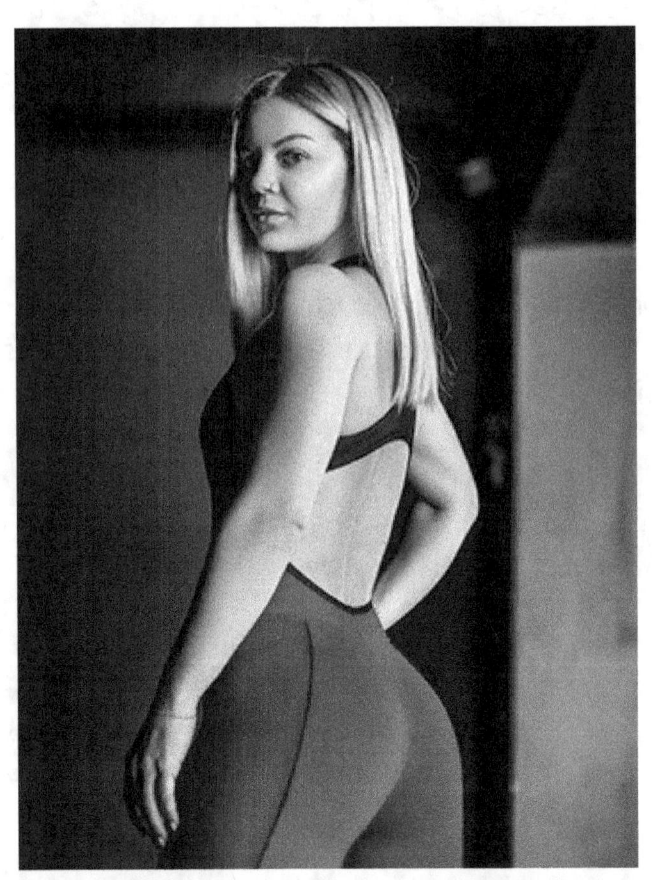

TABLE OF CONTENTS

3.1.	The shin. Raising the body on the socks.

3.2.	Quadriceps (front of the thigh). Squats for the quadriceps.

3.3.	A deep squat for the buttocks and the back of the thigh.

3.4.	Direct lunges in front of you.

3.5.	Sidelong lunges.

3.6.	Raising the pelvis, lying. The bridge is lying down.

3.7.	Gluteal Bridge with lifting one leg up.

3.8.	Lead one foot up from a kneeling position.

3.9.	Lifting the pelvis, sitting.

3.10.	Lifting the body with pacing to the chair, pulling the leg back.

3.11.	We stand against the wall and removal of the leg back.

3.12.	Lead legs to the side, on his knees.

3.13.	Breeding legs, lying on the floor

3.14.	Traction on bent legs.

3.15.	Thrust on one leg.

3.16.	Deep squatting, with a wide setting of the legs.

3.17.	Side steps in sitting position.

3.18.	Lunges back diagonally.

3.19.	Lunges to the sides, with wide stance.

3.20.	Leaving legs. Stand with support.

CHAPTER 1. What is the gluteal muscle? And how to make them elastic?

1.1. What is the buttocks?

These are three muscles - a large, medium and small gluteal. These three muscles form a beautiful and round women's ass. We will not go into anatomical knowledge with you. Since our book is created for ease of understanding - how to make elastic buttocks and make the legs slim at home. More often than not, girls around the world are concerned with the question - how to make an ass? How to pump it up, so that the skin does not hang? And how to remove the so-called "ears"?

1.2. What do we need to implement our plans?

Most importantly, we will need our desire. 25 minutes a day, from the props fit fitness mat or just a home mat. Also comfortable sportswear.

1.3. When is it better to do? And when it is already possible to start training?

It is better to do it every two days at the same time. We offer to do exercises in the morning. And to start training, you can right now, after reading these lines, so as not to put off a beautiful ass in the "later".

1.4. <u>And the last tip.</u>

Before you start the exercises - set a goal, 30 days to do this homework regularly and record your results. The easiest way to fix progress is to take a photo "before" and do a bi-weekly photo in the same position. And of course measurements. Take measurements of your body at the beginning of the training path. Girth of buttocks. Hip girth. Waist circumference. And we begin...

CHAPTER 2. Balanced nutrition. A key role.

2.1. "We are what we eat."

I think everyone is familiar with this famous phrase.
An important role in our training will be food. Everyone
knows that a healthy diet is the key to success, but not all
adhere to a balanced diet. What does balanced nutrition
mean when your body gets the right amount of protein,
fat and carbohydrates?

According to statistics, 70 percent of the world's
population neglects proteins in their diet. I'll explain what it
means. Most people eat a piece of meat or fish a day,
they can eat a little more potatoes or other side dishes in
the evening after work and in the morning, they drink
coffee with a croissant. If you count calories, then with this
diet, you will get a maximum of 1000-1200 calories, which
is an insanely small amount for the average person.

2.2. **Protein.**

Let's start with the protein. What is protein? Protein is an important building material of our body. From it consists, each cell body, it is included in all tissues and organs.

And now ask yourself a question - how often do you eat protein foods? If the answer you thought a long time and could not calculate how many times you ate protein for yesterday, then be sure you eat it a little.

How much protein do we need? 1 -2g per 1kg of body weight - it will be enough for your body to get the desired amino acids and build healthy cells, and even more so build a beautiful ass.

2.3. **Fats.**

Fats are a separate story. All people are afraid to eat fats and think that it is because of them that we have an imperfect weight. In fact, for metabolism in the body fats are very necessary. Fats are - saturated and non-saturated. Saturated fats - consider animal fats, unsaturated - vegetable. How not to twist, but these two kinds of fats are somehow needed by our body for metabolic processes. The main thing is not to overdo it. Our body needs fatty acids, such as Omega 3. They can be obtained either in its pure form or bought in a pharmacy.

Or eat fish and thus replenish the stores of fats in your body. It is also worth remembering that we definitely need to add to the salads different oils - olive, linseed, sesame and so on. They also contain many useful fatty acids. BUT the most important item is trans fats. This vegetable oil after frying - if to explain in simple words. That is, you need to minimize the use of oils during the frying of products and do not heat the oil.

2.4. <u>Carbohydrates.</u>

Carbohydrates - there are fast and slow. Slow - because their assimilation is long. Fast - because they are very quickly absorbed by our body and supply our cells with sugar, which contributes to a sharp rise in insulin in the blood, and of course can lead to fatness. Slow carbohydrates, in turn, supplement our body with enough vitamins and elements and saturation takes a long time and we do not feel hungry, like after fast food after half an hour. For example: fast carbohydrates - sugar, bakery products, dried fruits, chocolate, banana, carbonated water and juices, etc. Slow - different types of cereals, whole grains, vegetables, rice, etc.

2.5. <u>The result.</u>

We try to make our diet as rich as possible useful products, clean and not subject to severe heat treatment. To begin with, let's remove from the diet products such as bread, bars, chocolates, carbonated water and fried in oil products, as well as French fries and various sweets and biscuits.
In more detail about food we will talk in our next book.
Now we will dwell on exercises for the buttocks and legs.

CHAPTER 3. Training.

3.1. **The shin. Raising the body on the socks.**

- The number of repetitions is 20 times.
- The essence of the exercise - we lift our body to the socks, standing on the width of the shoulders. As shown in the photo.

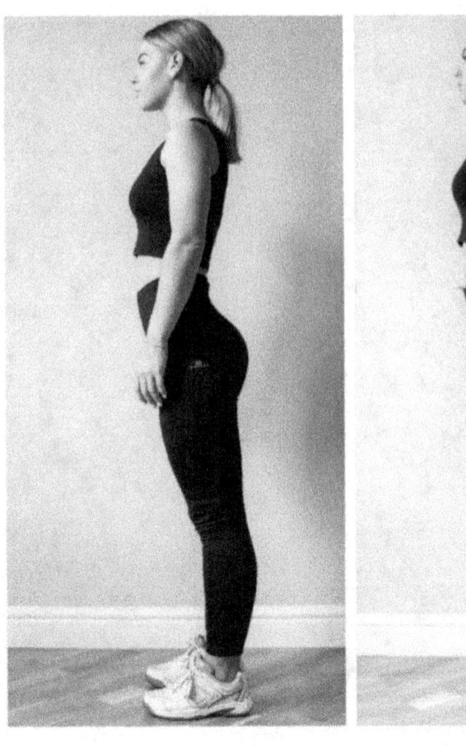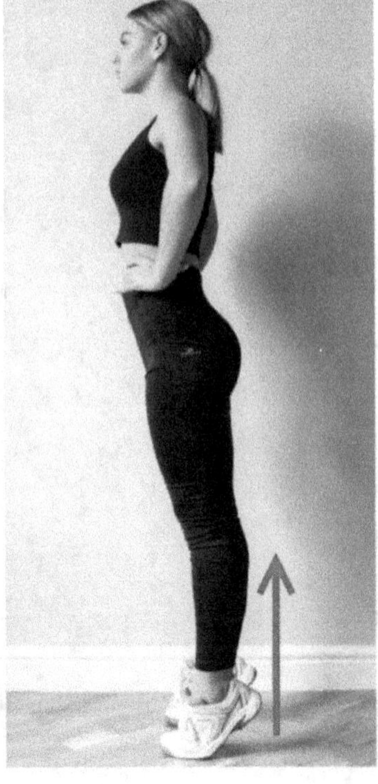

3.2. <u>Quadriceps (front of the thigh). Squats for the quadriceps.</u>

* The number of repetitions is 20 times.
* The essence of the exercise - we stand on level legs, legs are located on the width of the shoulders. While doing squats, pull the pelvis back as far as possible, while keeping an eye on the knees that should not go beyond the socks. If it is difficult to imagine the right technique, try to face the wall, the socks as close to the wall as possible, and take the pelvis back, while your knees will be fixed against the wall, so you will understand the essence of the exercise. As shown in the photo.

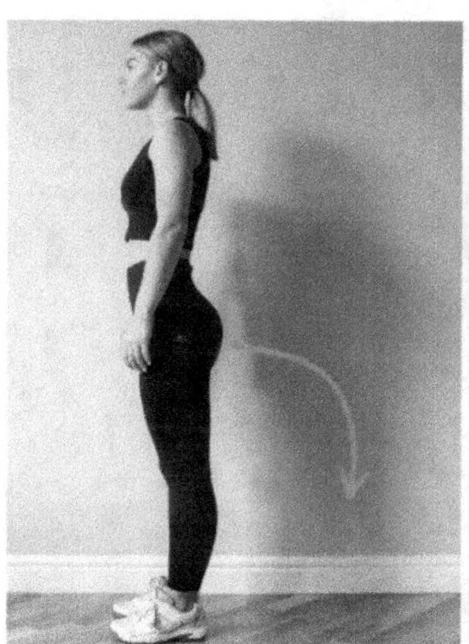 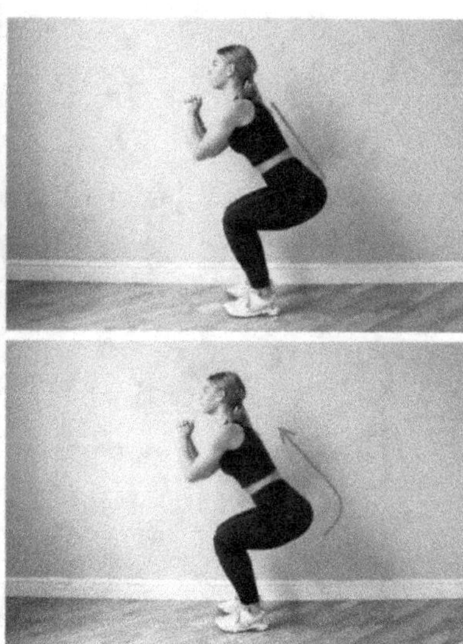

3.3. <u>A deep squat for the buttocks and the back of the thigh.</u>

• The number of repetitions is 20 times.
• The essence of the exercise - the setting of the legs - is wide, the socks are directed to the sides. The essence of the squat is the same as in the first exercise, only in this case we stretch the gluteus and hamstrings (thigh biceps). Maximum retraction of the pelvis back, making sure the correct position of the knees. Remember, your knees should not extend beyond toes, otherwise there is a variant of the knee injury. As shown in the photo.

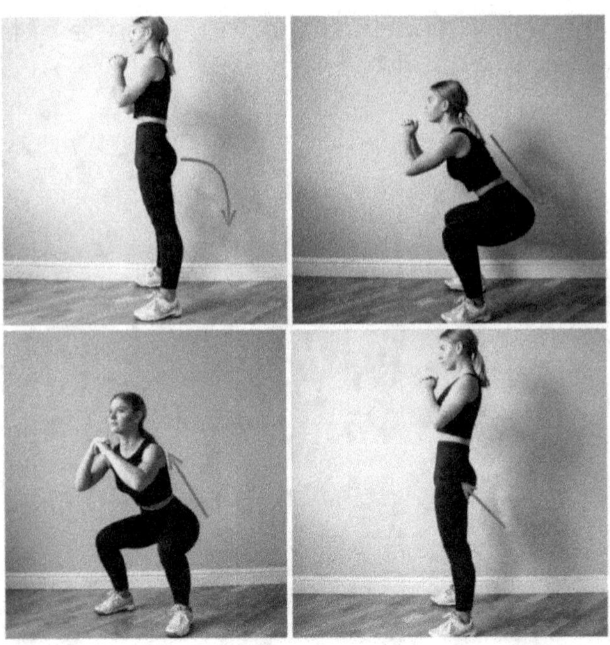

3.4. <u>Direct lunges in front of you.</u>

• The number of repetitions is 20 times.

• The essence of the exercise - We stand exactly, legs parallel to each other. (As shown in the photo). When performing the exercise, the center of gravity should be shifted to the front leg with an emphasis on the heel. Rise from squat and return to the starting position. Do the same exercise and the second leg with the same number of repetitions.

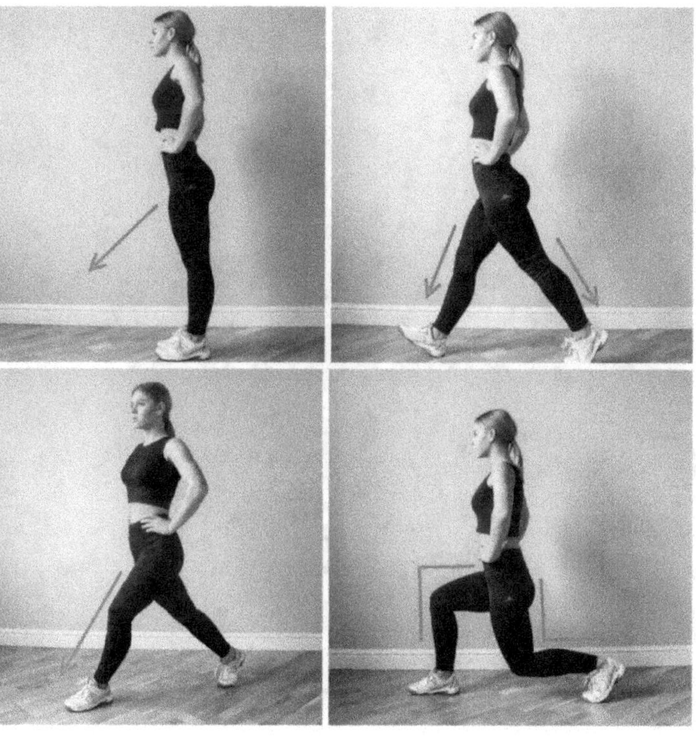

3.5. Sidelong lunges.

• The number of repetitions is 20 times.

• The essence of the exercise - We stand exactly, legs parallel to each other. From standing position, we make a wide step forward with one foot diagonally, so that we have a right angle (as shown in the photo). When performing the exercise, the center of gravity should be shifted to the front leg with an emphasis on the heel. Rise from squat and return to the starting position. Do the same exercise and the second leg with the same number of repetitions

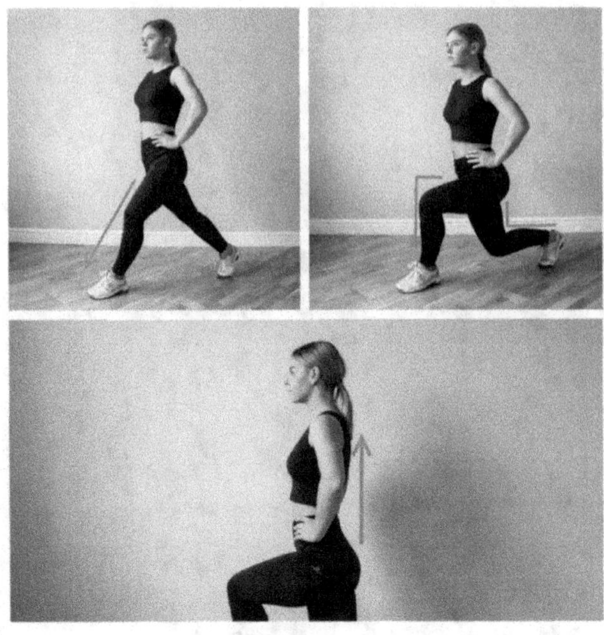

• The number of repetitions is 20 times.
• The essence of the exercise is the initial position of lying on the back. The arms are straight and are located along the body. Palms on the floor, knees bent:

-Lift the buttocks up above the floor, firmly resting their feet on the floor;

-stay in this position for two seconds and lower the pelvis;

-not touching the floor with the buttocks.

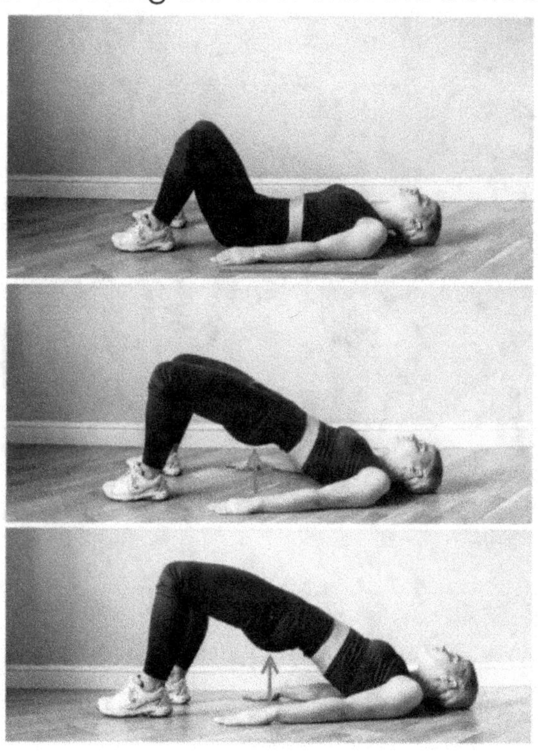

3.7. <u>Gluteal bridge with lifting one leg up.</u>

- The number of repetitions is 20 times.
- The essence of the exercise is the initial position of lying on the back. Arms straight alongside the body. Palms on the floor, one leg bent at the knee. The second leg is straight, stretched up; Push the leg up, thereby clamping the buttocks.
- When pushing the leg upwards, we stop for a second.

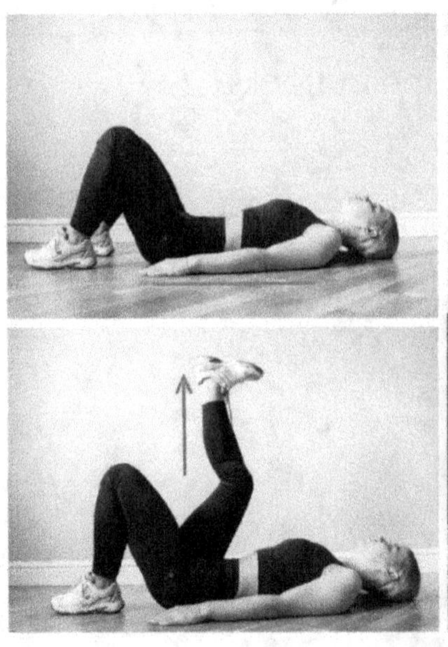

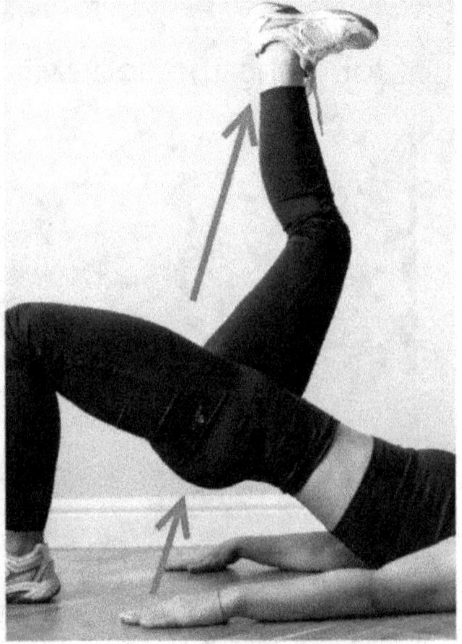

3.8. Lead one foot up from a kneeling position.

• The number of repetitions is 20 times.
• The essence of the exercise - We stand on all fours (as in the photo), we push each leg up one by one, put the accent on the heel, and push the leg out with the heel. The back is flat at this point and flexes slightly. We hold the leg for 2 seconds in the upper position.

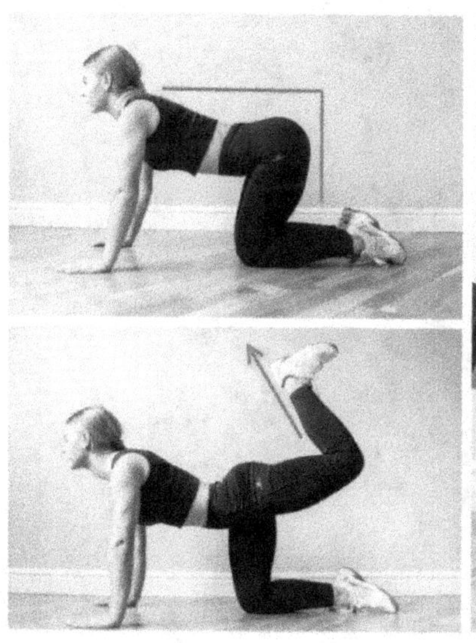
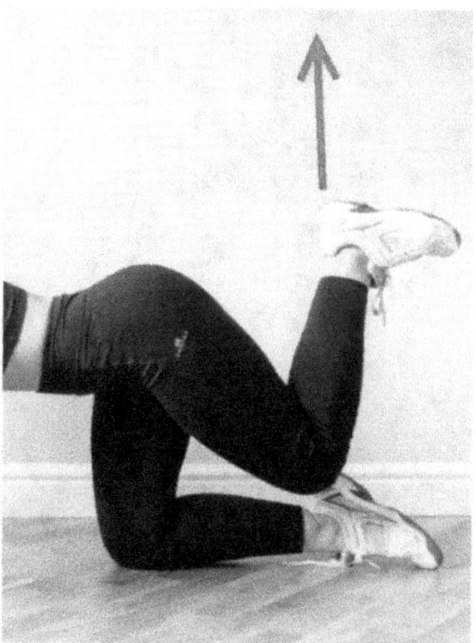

3.9. Lifting the pelvis, sitting.

• The number of repetitions is 20 times.
• The essence of the exercise - We sit on our knees, legs slightly wider than the hips. Lift the body up and hold the buttocks as tight as possible (as shown in the photo).

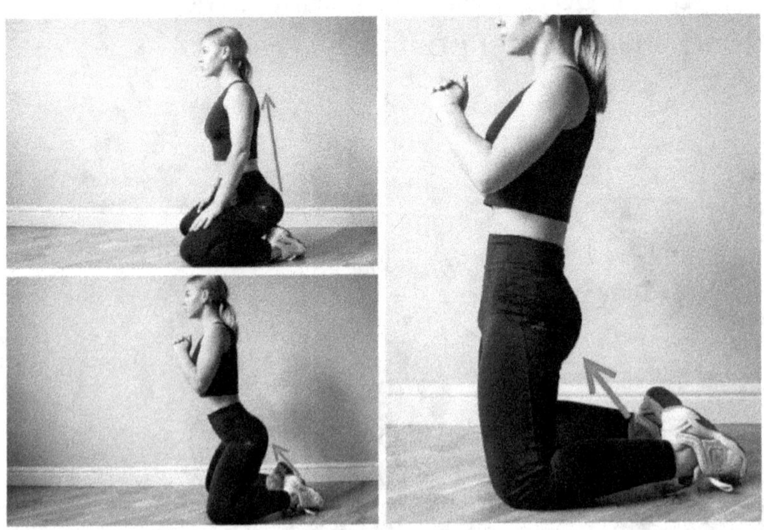

3.10. Lifting the body with pacing to the chair, pulling the leg back.

• The number of repetitions is 20 times.
• The essence of the exercise - the starting position - standing in front of the chair (curbstone), we step on a chair, the back is even. In the standing position on the chair, we remove the leg back, thereby straining the buttocks. (As shown in the photo).

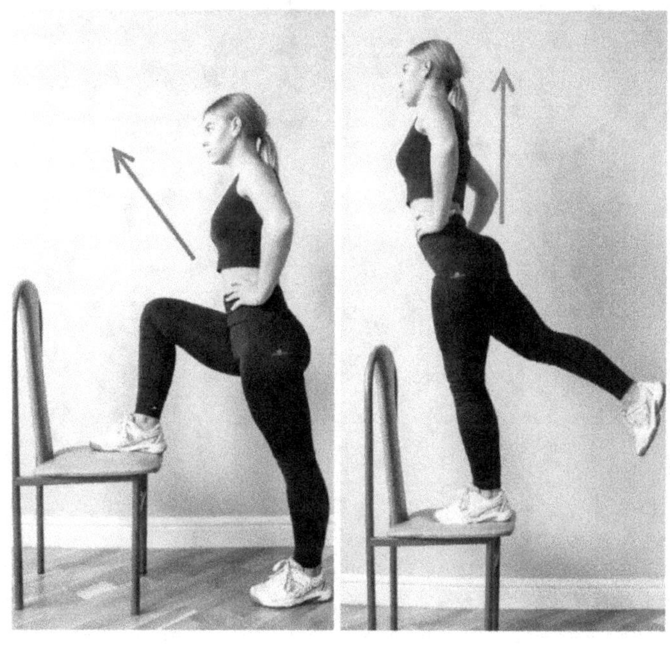

3.11. We stand against the wall and removal of the leg back.

- The number of repetitions is 20 times.
- The essence of the exercise - the starting position - we stand with the support at the wall. Take your foot back, clamping the buttocks for 2 seconds (as shown in the photo). Then we change the leg and do the same.

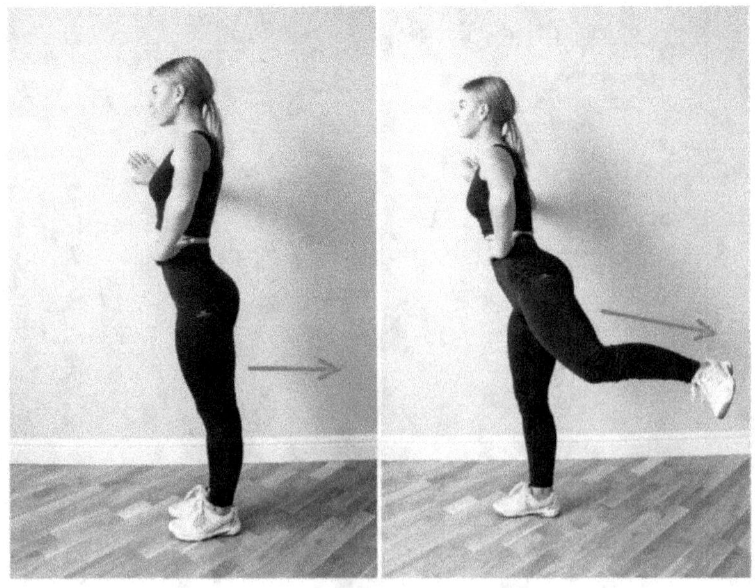

3.12. Lead legs to the side, on his knees.

• The number of repetitions is 20 times.
• The essence of the exercise - the starting position
- we stand on all fours, the back is even. The leg
bent at the knee is set aside, thereby training the
lateral surface of the buttocks and thighs.

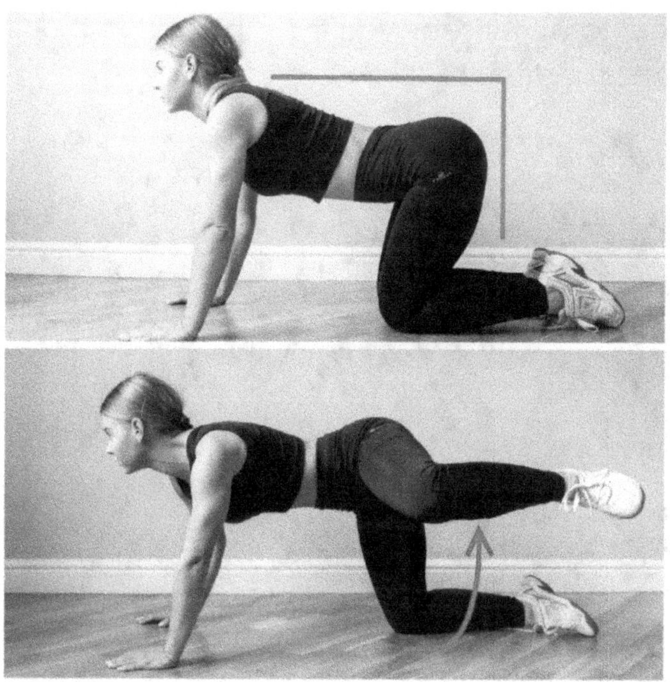

3.13. Breeding legs, lying on the floor.

• The number of repetitions is 20 times.
• The essence of the exercise - the starting position - we stand on all fours, the back is even. Move aside the leg, in a bent position (as shown in the photo), thereby you train the side of the buttocks and thighs.

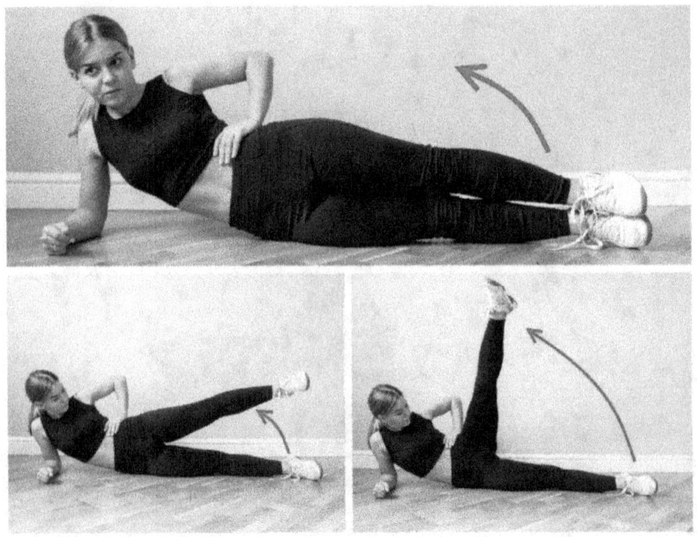

3.14. Traction on bent legs.

• The number of repetitions is 20 times.
• The essence of the exercise - the starting position - stand on the half-bent legs. Take the pelvis back as far as possible, lowering your hands along the body. Imagine that someone is pulling your hands on the buttocks. Knees should not extend beyond the toes. Your task is not to sit down, but to pull your buttocks back as far as possible, stretching the back surface of the thigh.

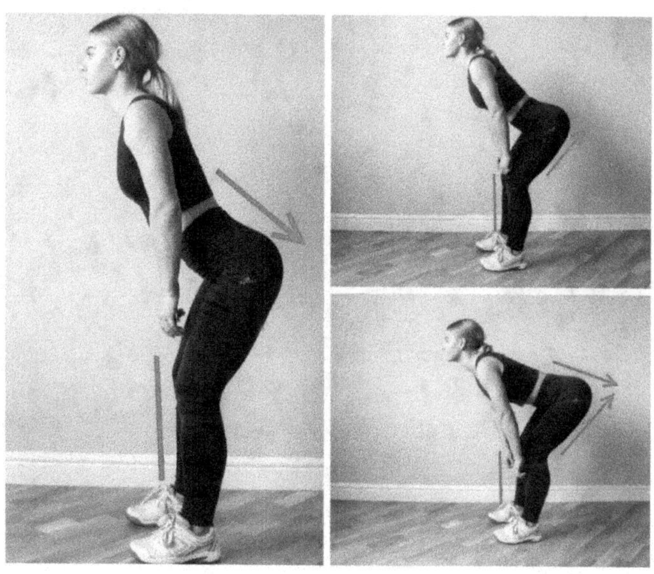

3.15. Thrust on one leg.

• The number of repetitions is 20 times.
• The essence of the exercise - the starting position - standing exactly on the legs. You can perform the exercise standing against the wall (as shown in the photo). Pull the leg backwards, making the body tilt. Then change your leg and do 20 repetitions again.

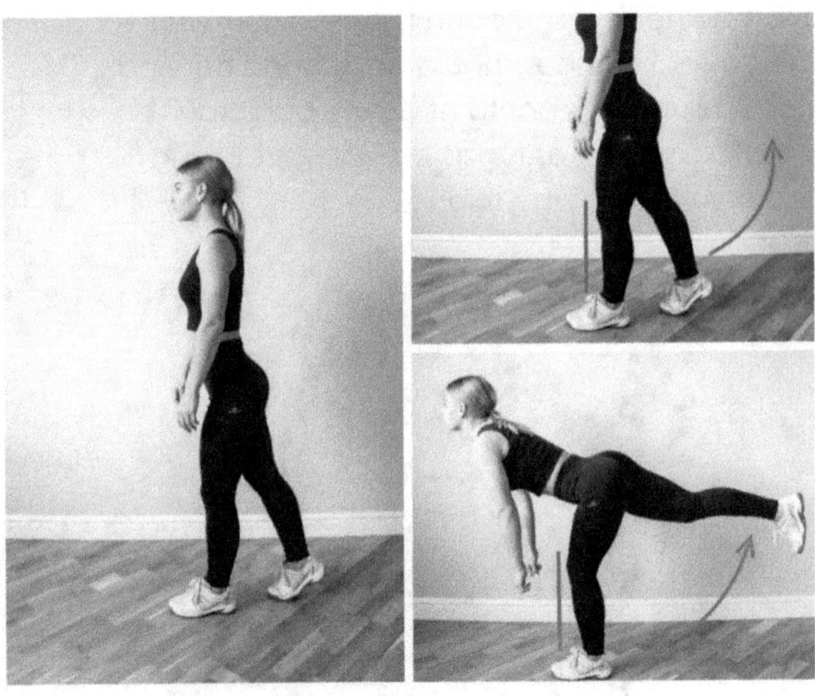

<u>3.16. Deep squatting, with a wide setting of the legs.</u>

- The number of repetitions is 20 times.
- The essence of the exercise - the legs are set wide, the socks are unfolded in the sides. Squat as deeply as possible. In the hands, you can take some heavy object, if you are easy without weight. When you return to the starting position - pinch the maximum buttocks.

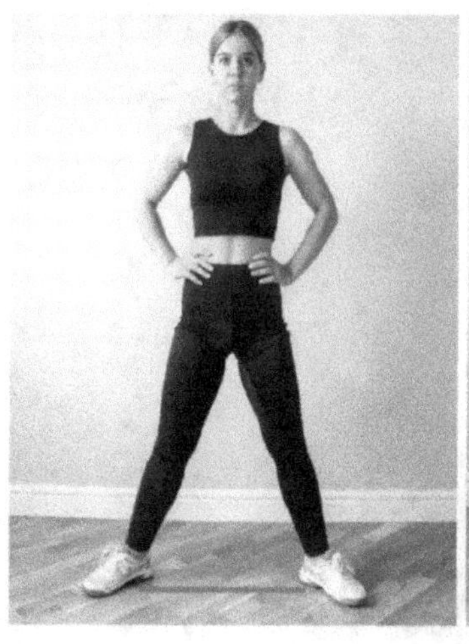 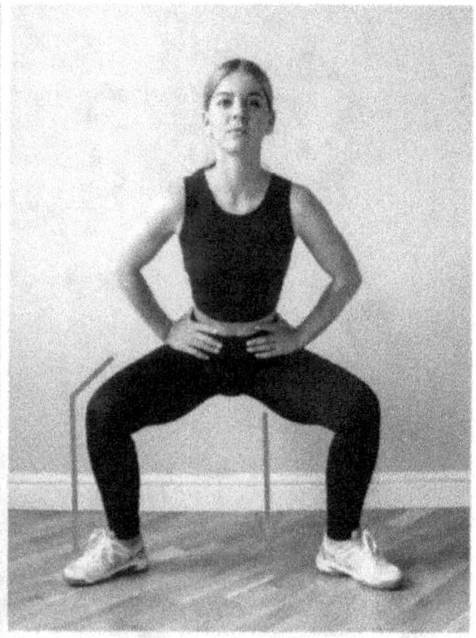

3.17. Side steps in sitting position.

• The number of repetitions is 20 times.
• The essence of the exercise - the legs are set slightly wider than the hips, squat and start moving to the side. Side steps should be 20 with each leg. Try to keep your back straight.

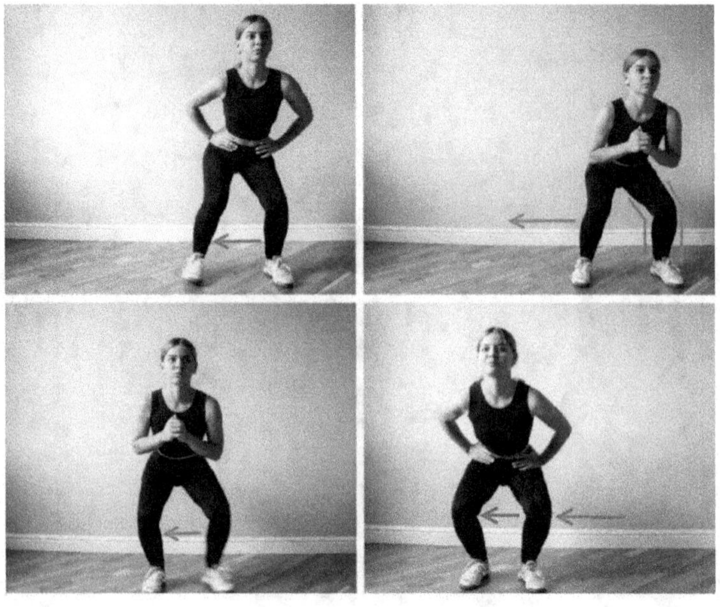

3.18. Lunges back diagonally.

- The number of repetitions is 20 times.
- The essence of the exercise - the starting
position - stand on your feet. Make a wide
step back diagonally, forming again a
straight angle with the knees. Focus shift to
the heel of the foot, which remains in front.
When you lift the body to its original position,
lean on the heel.

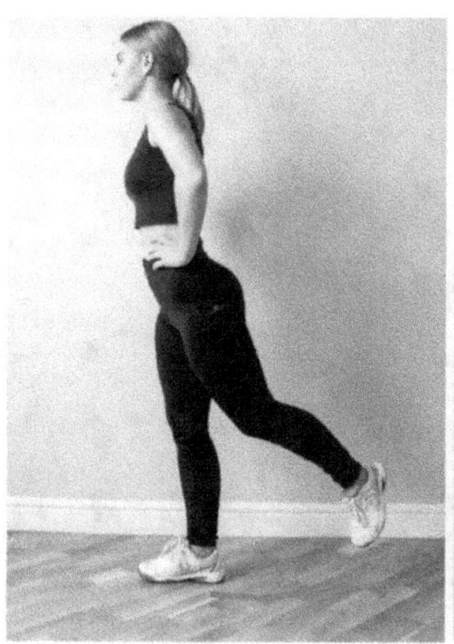 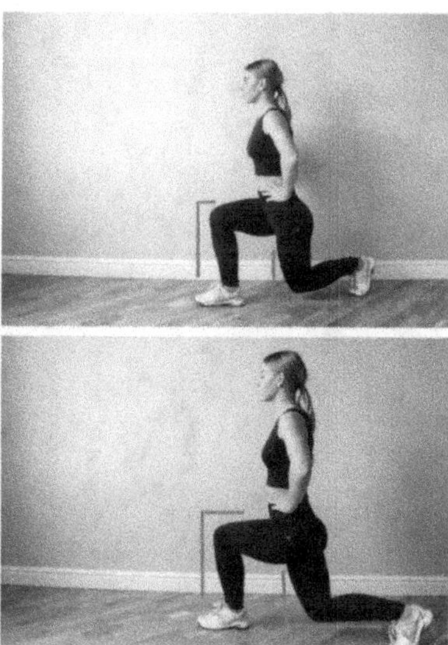

3.19. Lunges to the sides, with wide stance.

- The number of repetitions is 20 times.
- The essence of the exercise - the starting position - a wide setting of the legs. Make lunges to the side as shown in the photo. This exercise tightens the inner thighs.

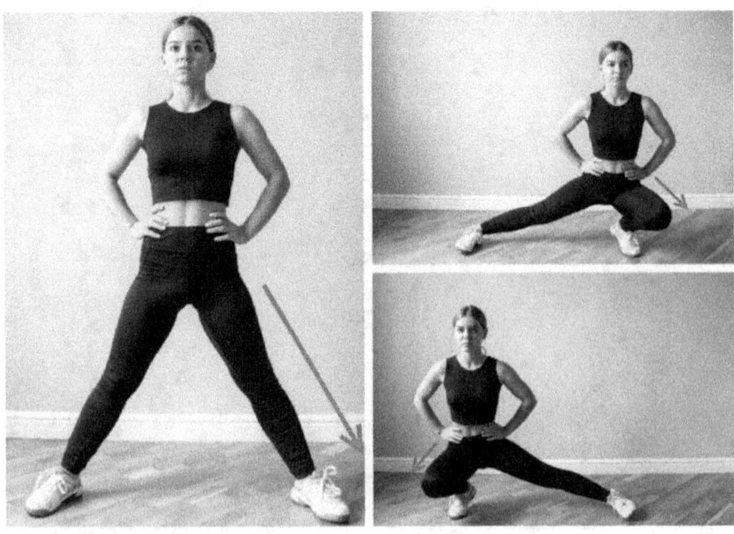

<u>3.20.</u> <u>Leaving legs. Stand with support.</u>

- The number of repetitions is 20 times.
- The essence of the exercise - the
starting position - stand exactly on two
legs. Take one of the legs back,
clamping the buttocks (as shown in the
photo). Then change legs.

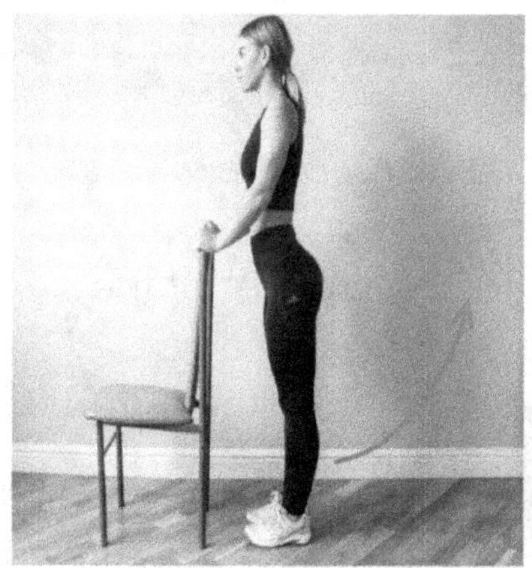 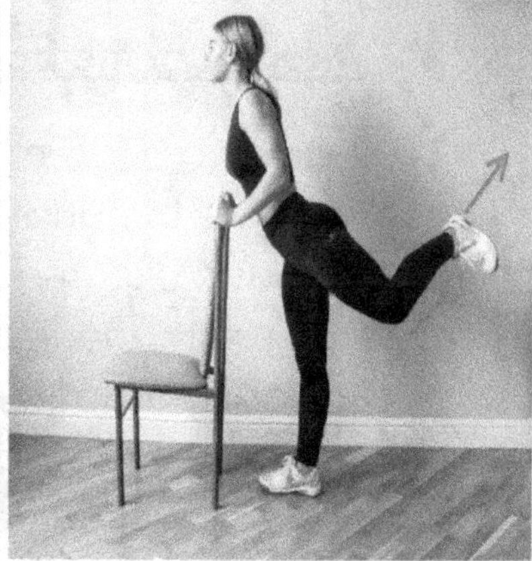

CHAPTER 4. What do "upper body" exercises include?

4.1. **Deltoid muscles - that is, shoulders.**

Deltoid muscles have three tufts. Why deltoid - because the shape of the bundles of the muscles of the shoulder has the form of a triangle, hence the name "Delta". Three beams are the front delta, middle and back. We will perform exercises for all the beams.

4.2. **Muscles of the back.**

The back is a huge muscle group. We will not disassemble the anatomical component; we will do basic exercises for the muscles of the back. Visually, the figure of the girls looks very beautiful, roughly speaking, in the form of an hourglass! In order for the figure to have this appearance, we will train the latissimus muscles of the back, and work to strengthen the muscular corset of the back as a whole.

4.3. <u>Hands.</u>

Weak Hands - the eternal problem of girls. In our book you will learn about triceps and biceps training. All the exercises and techniques of execution are shown in the photo, and you can exactly repeat them at home.

4.4. <u>Chest.</u>

We have chosen for you the most basic exercises on the pectoral muscles, so that you can pull up the lagging. Girls need this for a common muscular corset and even posture.

5.1.   Take your hands aside.

• The number of repetitions is 20 times.

• The essence of the exercise - we take a fitness gum, we become exactly with legs lightly bent at the knees. Our task is to spread our arms to the sides, so that the elbow looks upwards, and it is with the elbow that we set the motion (not with the brush, but with the elbow). This exercise can be called "pour water from the pitchers." Imagine that you have jugs in your hand and you need to pour water out of them.

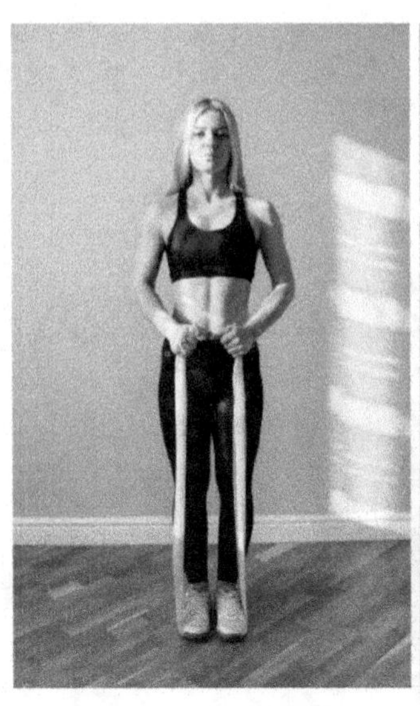
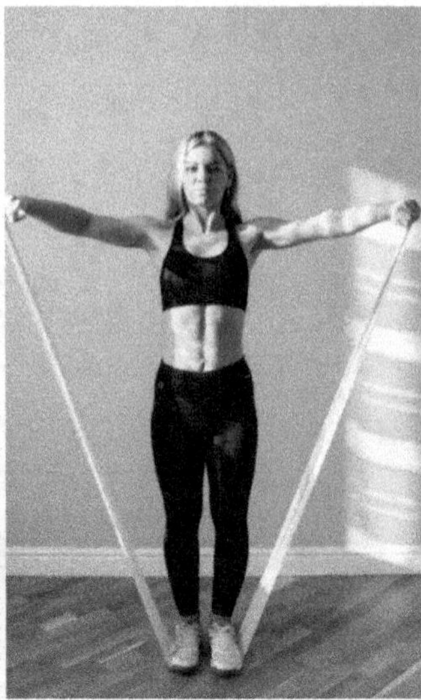

<u>5.2.</u> <u>Leading the arms to the front delta.</u>

- The number of repetitions is 20 times.
- The essence of the exercise - we take a fitness gum, stand on it exactly, legs bent at the knees. Bent arms in the elbows are removed in front of him, thus the front side of the shoulder works.

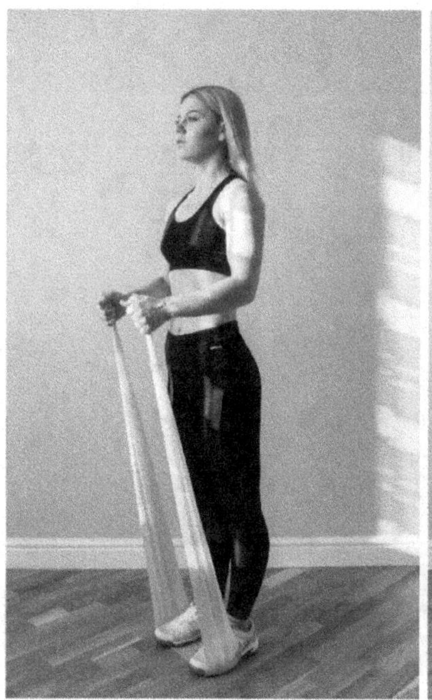 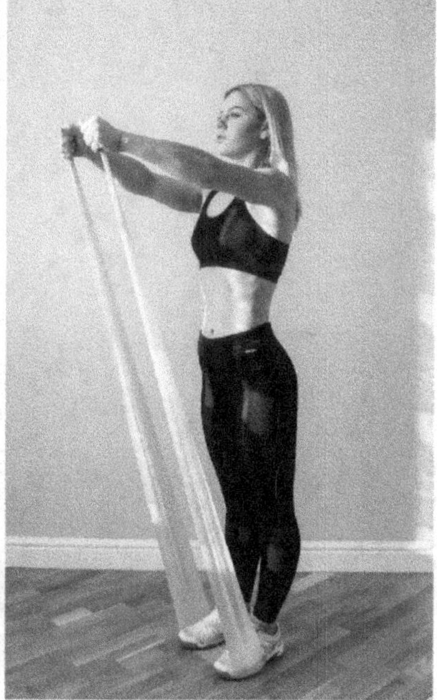

<u>5.3. Press standing. Exercise for the middle delta.</u>

- The number of repetitions is 20 times.
- The essence of the exercise - we take a fitness gum, stand on an elastic band with bent at the knees, hold the elastic band, as shown in the picture. We push hands upward, parallel to the body.

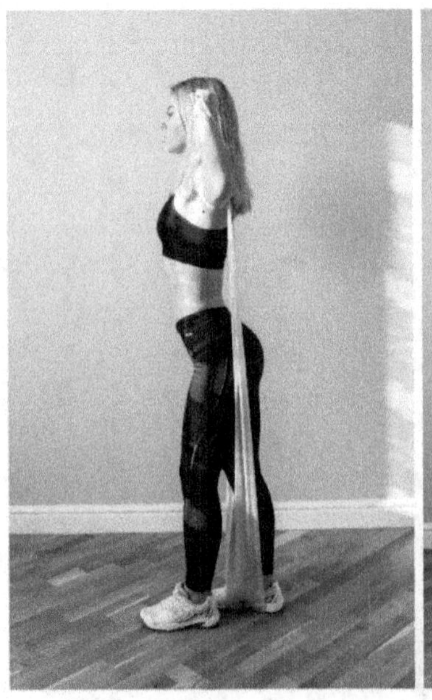 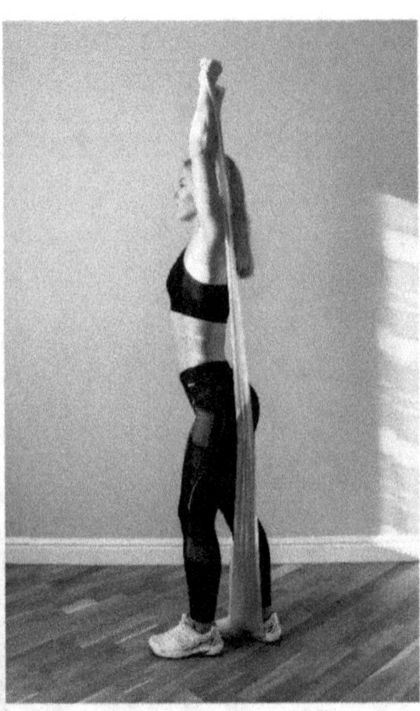

5.4. Thrust gum to the chin, exercise on the middle delta.

- The number of repetitions is 20 times.
- The essence of the exercise - we take a fitness gum, stand on an elastic band with bent at the knees, hold the elastic band, as shown in the picture. We step on the elastic with the two legs, pull the elastic band to the chin, so that the elbows are at the maximum at an angle.

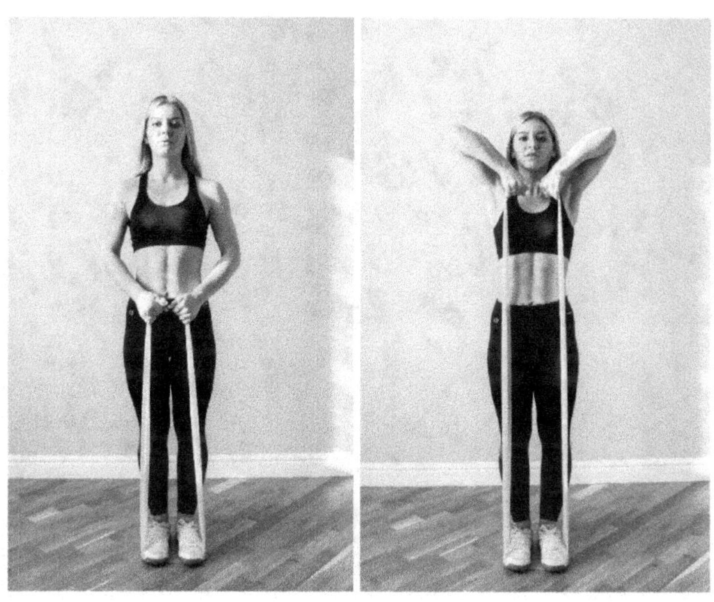

5.5. Exercise to the rear delta.

- The number of repetitions is 20 times.
- The essence of the exercise - you take a fitness gum, to become even with slightly bent legs. Pull the rubber band, as shown in the picture, pulling our hands apart, pulling our elbows to the ceiling. Thus, the posterior deltoid muscle is involved.

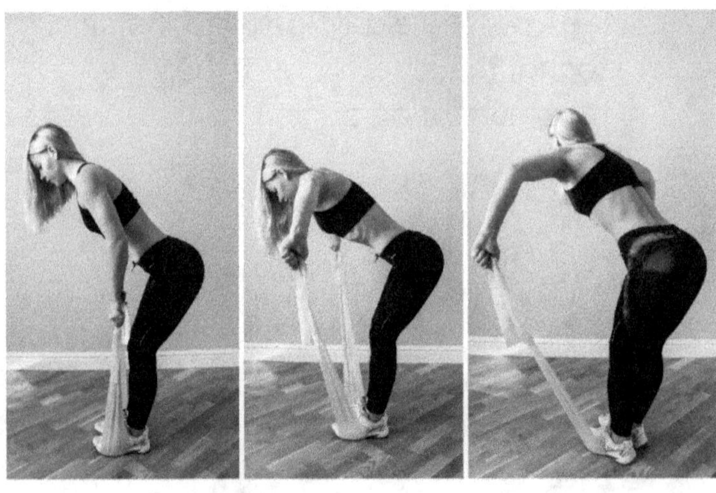

<u>5.6.</u>   <u>An exercise for the shoulders. we spread our hands in turns.</u>

- The number of repetitions is 20 times.
- The essence of the exercise - you take a fitness gum, to become even with slightly bent legs. Elbow looks at the ceiling. do the exercise as shown at the picture.

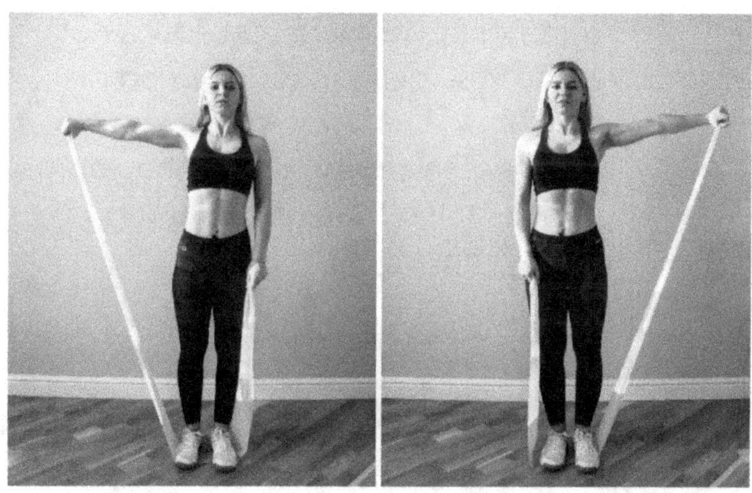

CHAPTER 6. Training. Arms.

6.1. <u>Biceps.</u>

- The number of repetitions is 20 times.
- The essence of the exercise - you take a fitness gum, to become even with slightly bent legs. Our task is not just to raise our hands and bend at the elbow, the task is to squeeze the biceps of the hand. Elbows should remain at the base of the trunk and do not move.

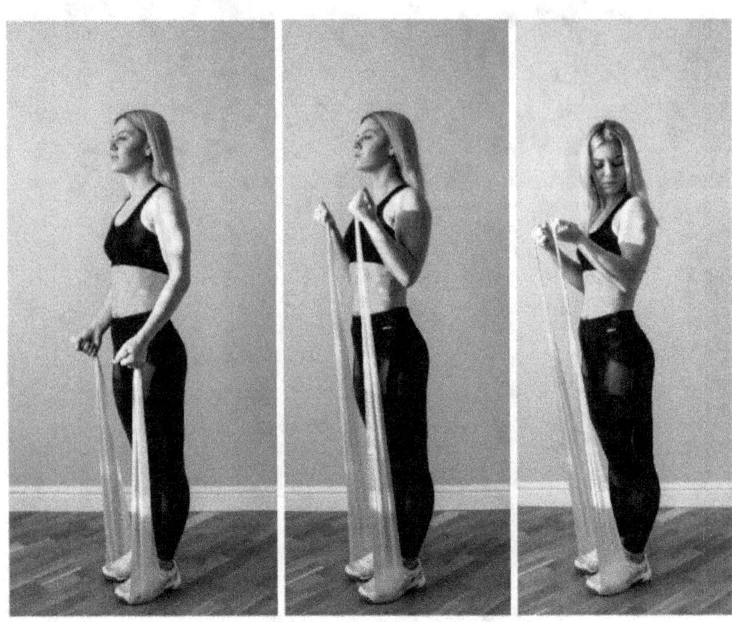

6.2. __The triceps.__

- The number of repetitions is 20 times.
- The essence of the exercise - you take a fitness gum, to become even with slightly bent legs. We have become on the elastic band with two legs. The body is tilted forward as shown in the figure, hands parallel to the body. Our task- is to take our hands to the starting position, while we are working triceps. Exercise is like skiing.

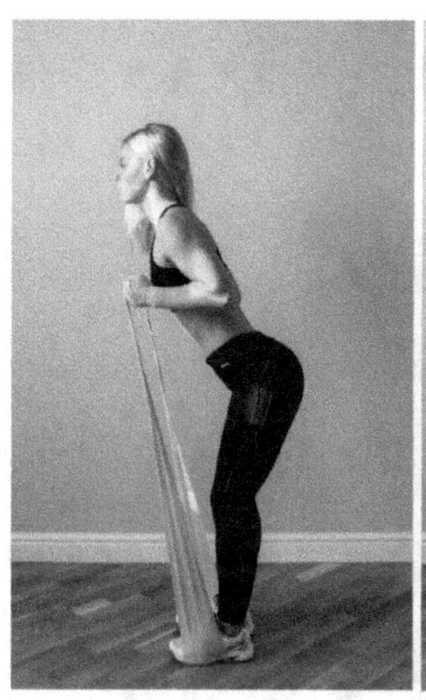
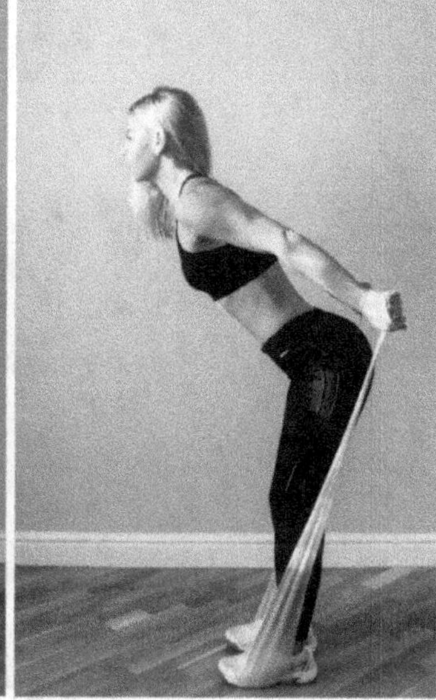

6.3.   **Push-up for triceps.**

- The number of repetitions is 20 times.
- The essence of the exercise - we lay down on the floor so that the hands are at the bottom of the body. the initial position of our body is a flat body, without sagging in the pelvis and on straight hands. perform the exercise as shown in the photo.

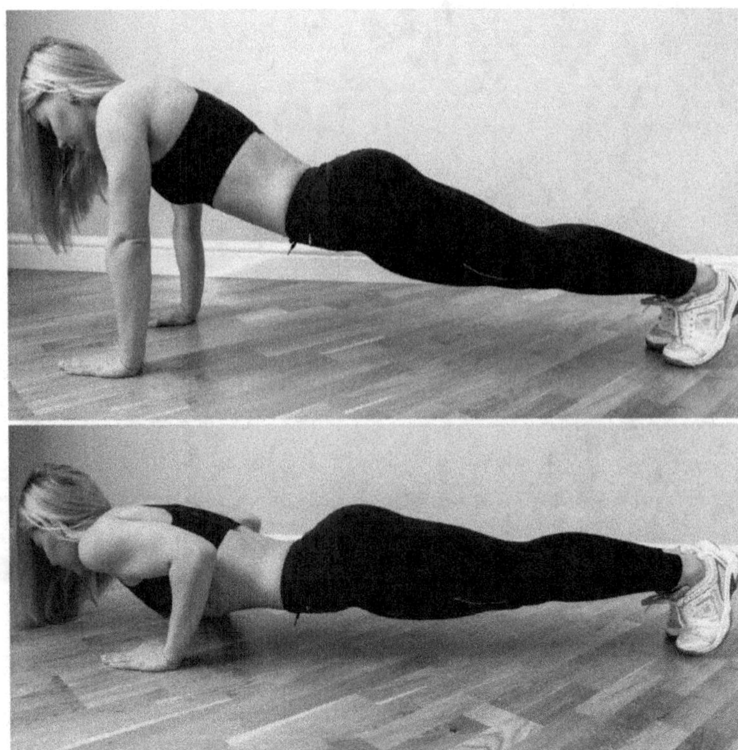

CHAPTER 7. Training. Chest.

7.1. <u>Push-ups for pectoral muscles.</u>

- The number of repetitions is 20 times.
- The essence of the exercise - the body is even, the arms are wider than the shoulders, our task is pressed from the floor. Perform the exercise as shown in the photo.

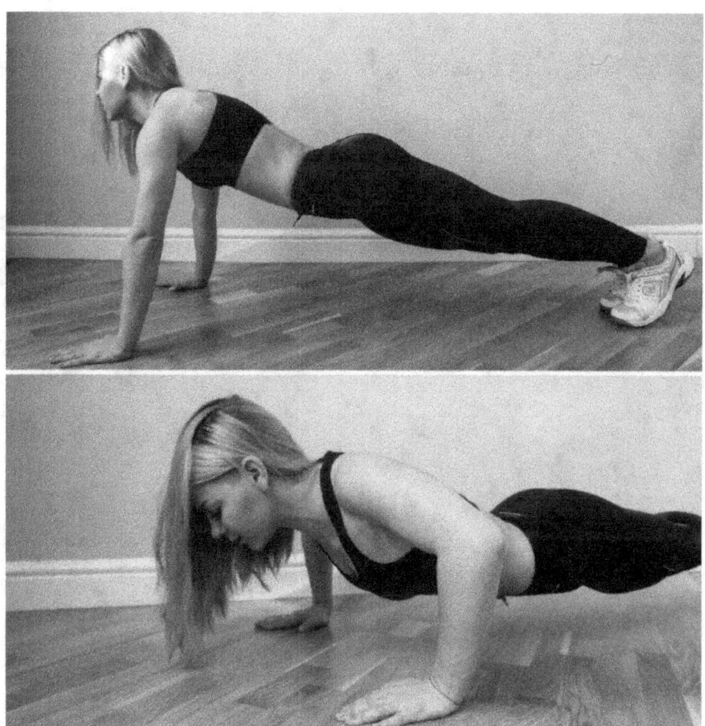

7.2. General exercise for the muscles of the chest.

- The number of repetitions is 20 times.
- The essence of the exercise - standing position. We take the rubber band by the center, as shown in the picture. Our task is to straighten our hands. We do this exercise intensively alternately changing hands.

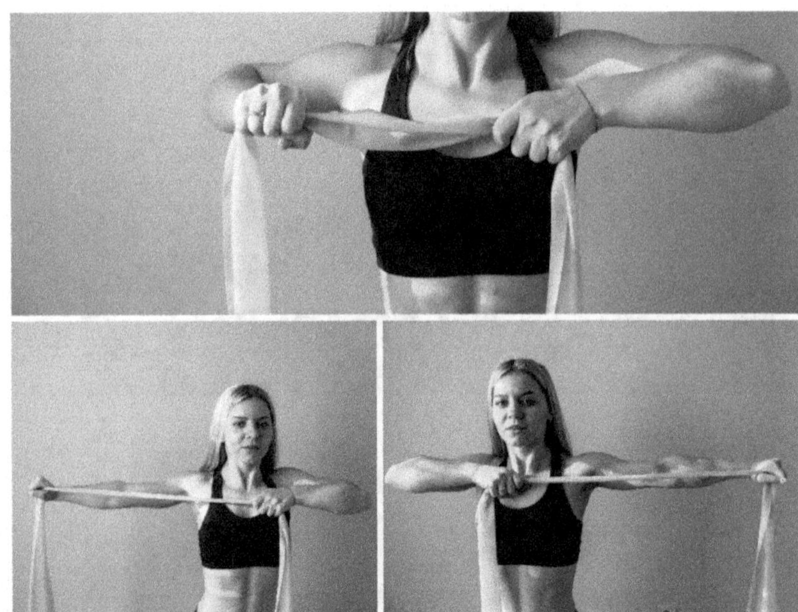

CHAPTER 8. Training. Back.

8.1. <u>Thrust gum to the body.</u>

- The number of repetitions is 20 times.
- The essence of the exercise - the initial position of "lunges". one leg in front. The back is slightly tilted forward. Our task is to pull the elastic band to the body, bring the shoulder blades together (as shown in the photo)

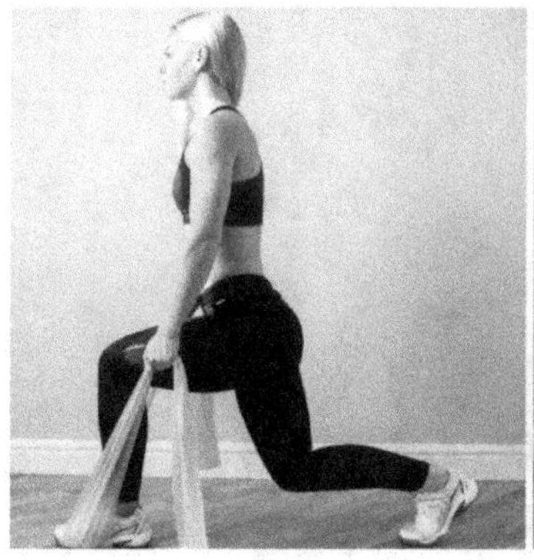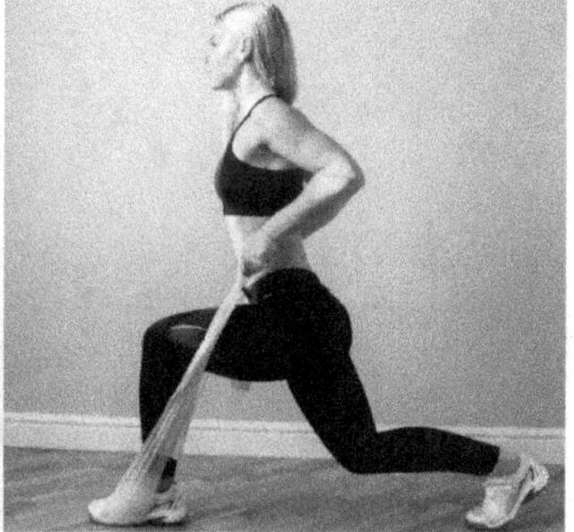

<u>8.2.</u>   <u>Pull of fitness gum from the sitting position.</u>

- The number of repetitions is 20 times.
- The essence of the exercise - the starting position of sitting with even legs. Rubber to the feet as shown in the photo. Our task is to pull the elastic band to the bottom of the abdomen and to unite shoulder blades. Do intensely 20 times.

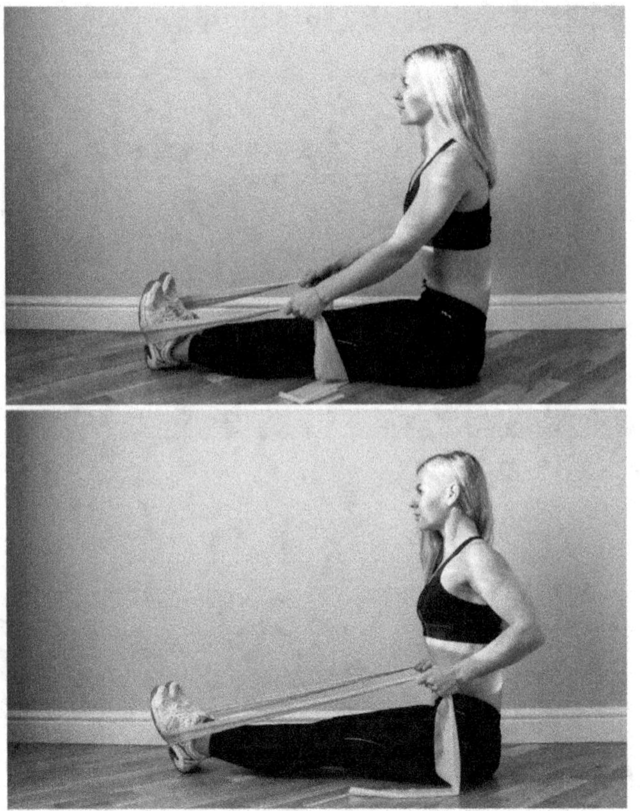

CHAPTER 9. Functional final exercise on the entire upper body.

- The number of repetitions is 20 times.
- The essence of the exercise is to do the so-called "cross". As it is shown on the picture. Cases intensively 20 times.

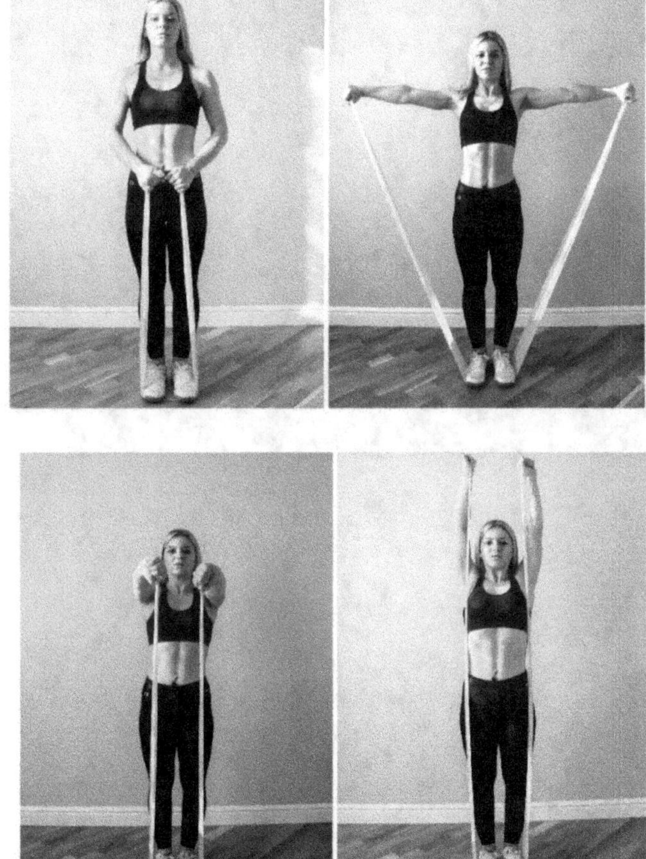

CHAPTER 10. Circular exercise on the joints. Warm-Up.

- This exercise you can perform as a warm-up, and at the end of the exercises as a hitch. The exercise warms up the joints well, and at the end of the exercise, it relaxes the joints well and stretches the ligaments. Execution is shown in the photo.

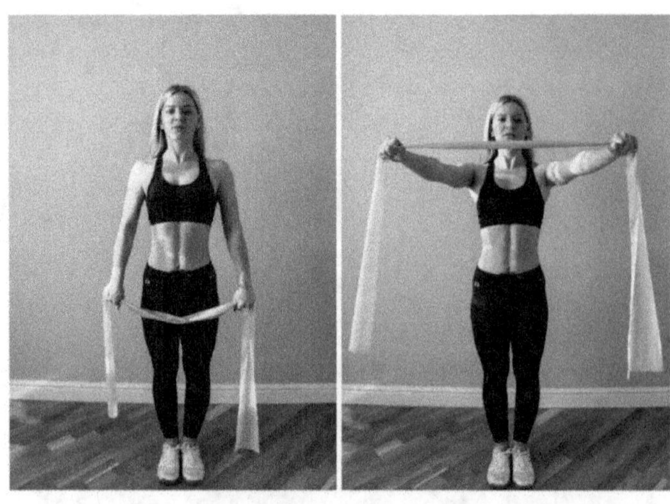

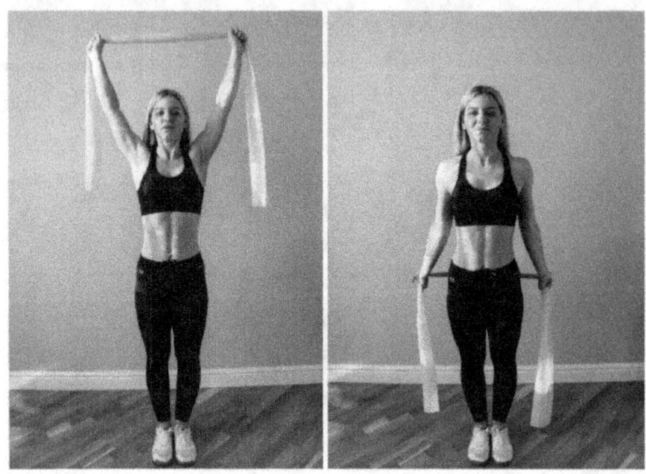

CHAPTER 11. What are the abdominal muscles?

11.1. Abdominal muscles. Structure.

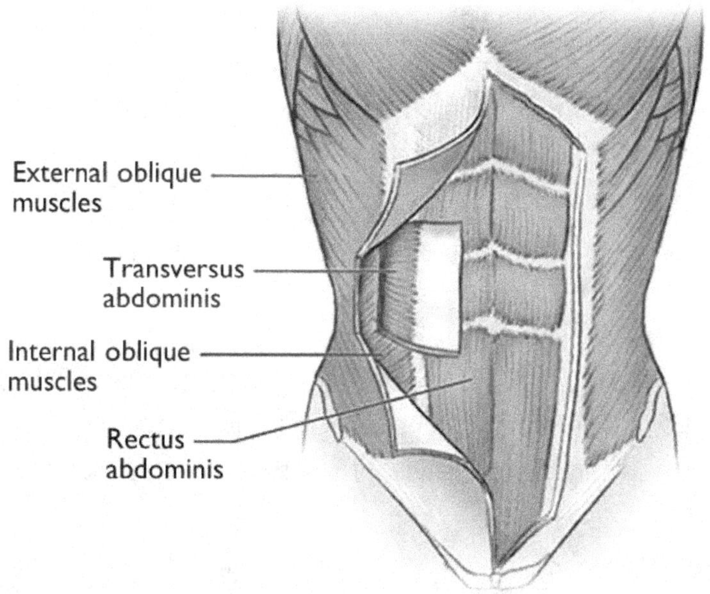

The abdominal muscles (press) consists of four main muscles: a rectus abdominis, an external oblique, and internal oblique and transverse muscle.

Let us examine in more detail.

The rectus abdominis muscle is the long muscle of the anterior wall of the abdominal cavity. It starts with the pubic comb, extends to the top of the abdomen and attaches to the ribs and sternum. The very "cubes" are formed when interrupted by the transverse tendon ligaments of the muscle fibers. What is the function of the real muscle? Function of flexing the human torso forward, also pulling the hips down and lifting the pelvis when the chest is fixed.

Outer oblique abdominal muscle. This muscle is the most extensive muscle on the abdomen, it is its fibers that go obliquely from the top down. Only the oblique muscle pulls our ribs down and bends the trunk. And with a simultaneous contraction of the left and right muscles, she lifts the pelvis, if the chest is strengthened. When unilateral reduction, oblique turning torso in the opposite direction.

The internal oblique muscle. The internal muscle is under the outer oblique muscle of the abdomen and forms the second layer of the abdominal wall. Internal oblique muscles are also responsible for flexing the body.

Transverse abdominal muscle. The transverse muscle forms the third layer of the muscles of the abdominal wall and is just the deepest. This muscle goes around the waist and placed horizontally. This set of muscles forms the abdominal press. The transverse muscle is responsible for turning the body in the sides around the axis, and also bends the trunk forward and sideways.

Exercises are presented in our third booklet, for example, do not impose. We also recommend choosing from 12 exercises for three or four and doing them regularly, changing them and alternating. Carrying out regularly and technically these exercises - you will succeed.

CHAPTER 12. Types of exercises. Options.

12.1. <u>Hull Lift (body).</u>

- The number of repetitions is 20 times.
- The essence of the exercise - Lying on the floor (rug), your task is to squeeze the muscles of the press, and then your body itself will rise. Our task is to squeeze the muscles well, it is not necessary to immediately touch the knees. Do Exercise on exhalation, as shown on the photo.

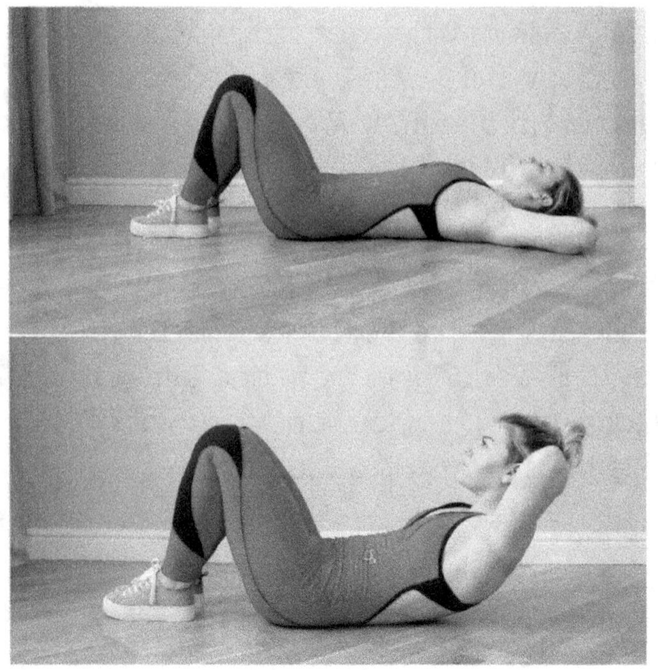

<u>12.2. Lifting the hull (hands on the diagonal, like a bicycle.</u>

* The number of repetitions is 20 times.
* The essence of the exercise - the starting position - lie on the floor. Our task is to touch the knees with our elbows. This exercise is similar to riding a bicycle. You take turns to touch the knees as you exhale, as shown in the figure.

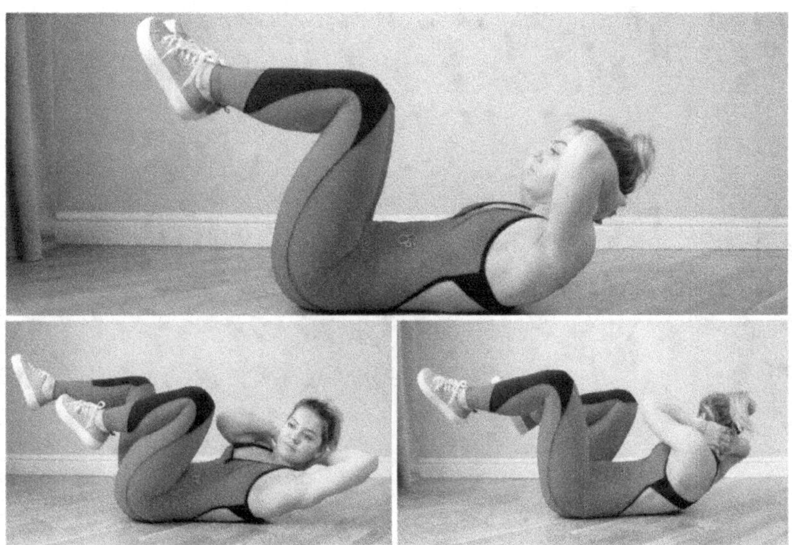

<u>12.3.</u>   <u>Lying, touch the heels.</u>

- The number of repetitions is 20 times.
- The essence of the exercise - your task is to touch alternately your feet (as shown in the photo), thus we are working on the oblique muscles of the press. The further you put the legs the more difficult it will be for you to reach and thereby you will improve your results.

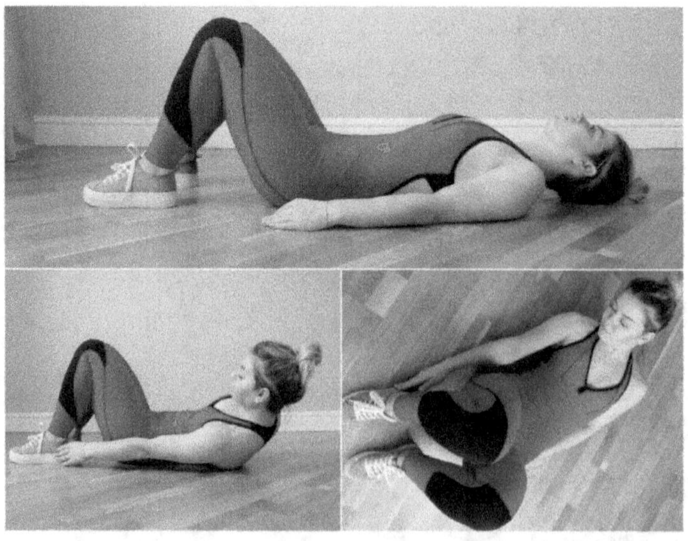

12.4. Exercise "Book".

- The number of repetitions is 20 times.
- The essence of the exercise - your task is to twist like a book (as shown in the photo). In this exercise all the abdominal muscles are involved and you can train this muscle group as cool as possible.

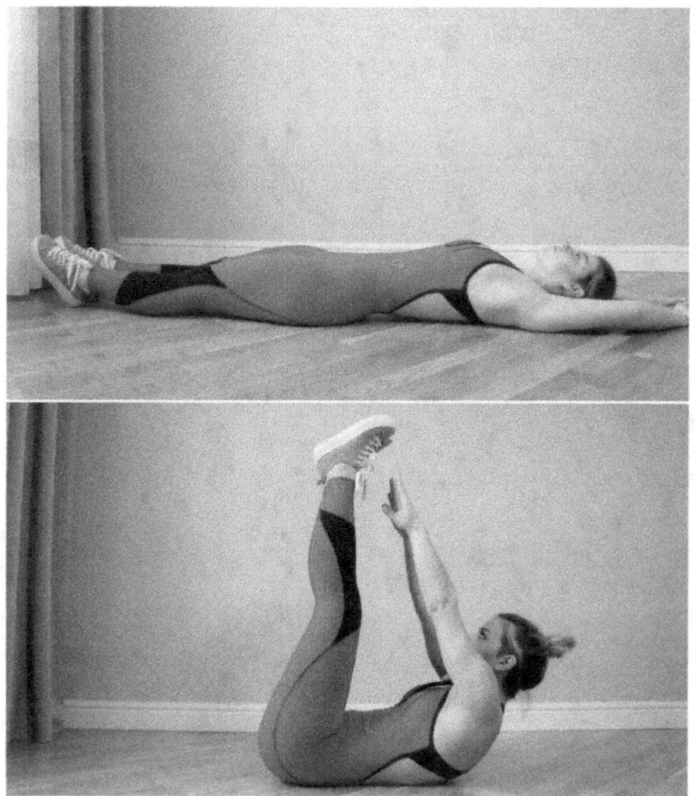

12.5. <u>Twisting of the body.</u>

- The number of repetitions is 20 times.
- The essence of the exercise - your feet are even and elevated. The task will alternately touch the feet with the palms. So-called body twisting.

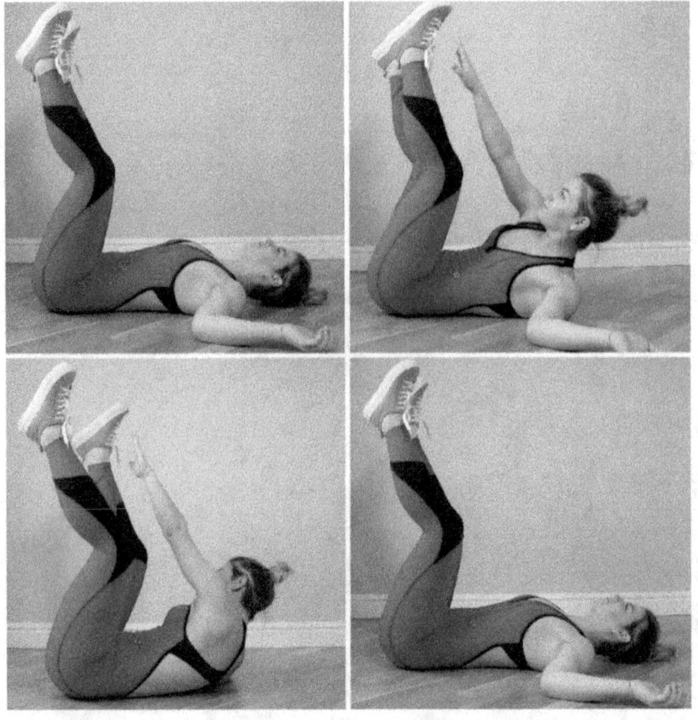

12.6. <u>Touch the toes, raised legs.</u>

- The number of repetitions is 20 times.
- The essence of the exercise - Another kind of twisting, or rather, lifting the hull. Your task is to keep your legs in one position (as shown in the photo) and climb up on exhalation, and touch both feet simultaneously. So we use all the muscles of our belly.

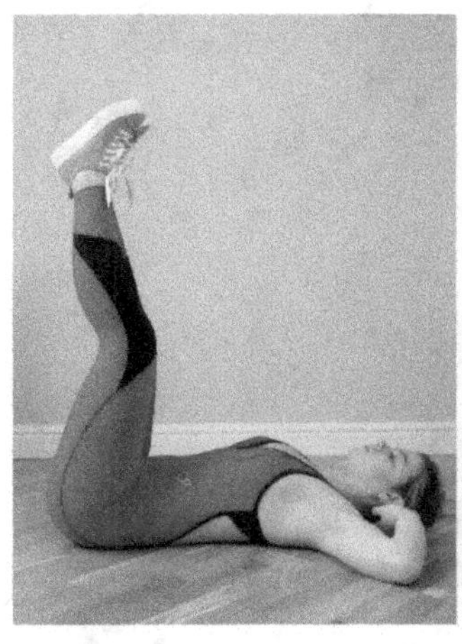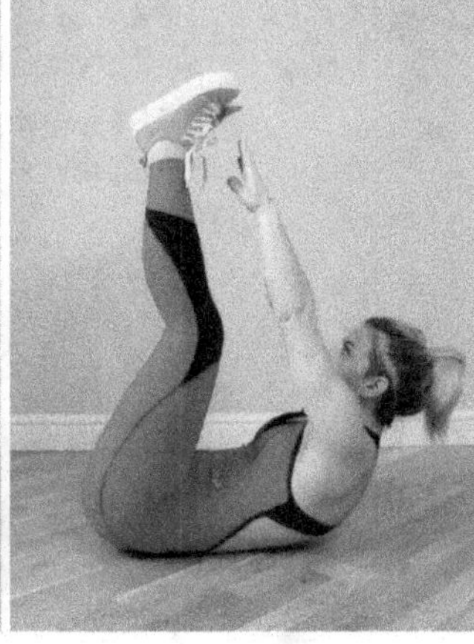

12.7. <u>Lifting the body, touching the socks.</u>

- The number of repetitions is 20 times.
- The essence of the exercise - take the starting position - lying on the floor, or on the mat. The legs are bent at the knees. Our task is to lift the body on exhalation. You must touch your feet with your hands.

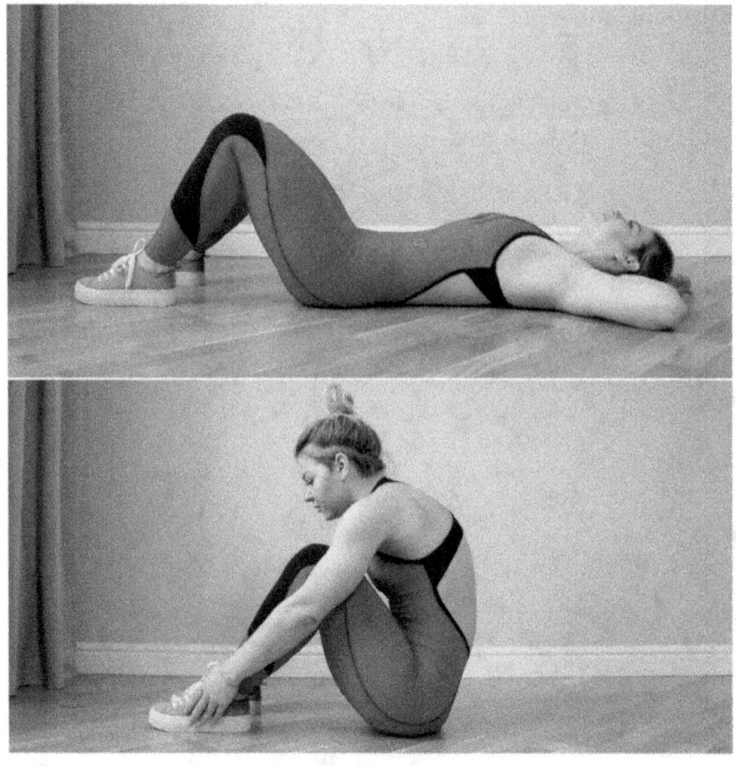

12.8. <u>Raising feet by 45 degrees.</u>

- The number of repetitions is 20 times.
- The essence of the exercise - We perform the exercise for the lower part of the press. We hold our legs practically at the same angle and alternately change them. Hands can be put under the buttocks, and then you will be more comfortable to work.

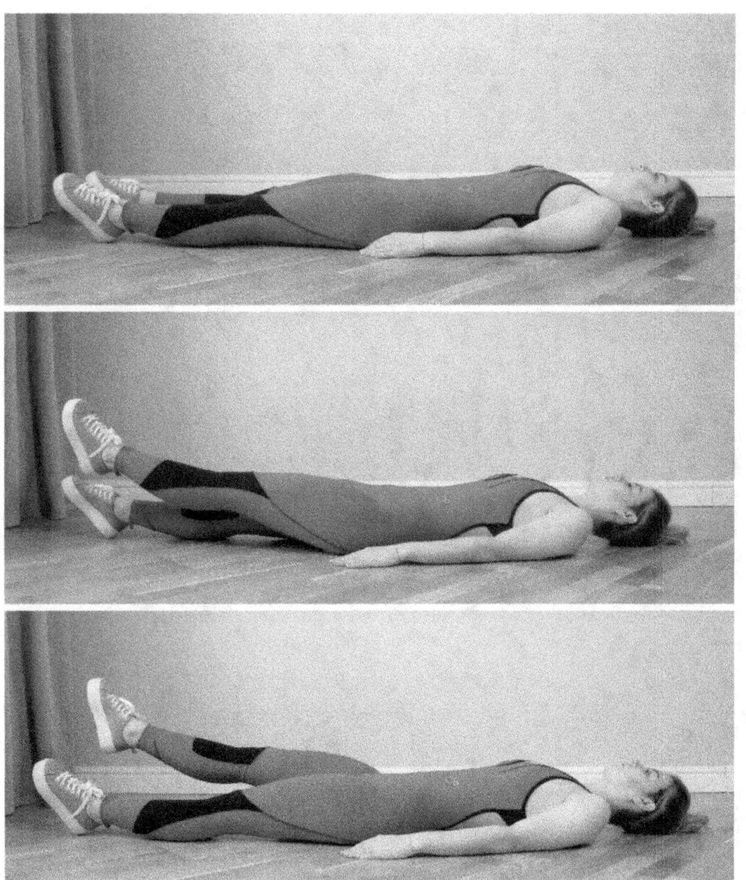

12.9. <u>**Torsion of the pelvis.**</u>

- The number of repetitions is 20 times.
- The essence of the exercise - we raise the pelvis and twist it on ourselves, while exhaling we perform the exercise. So we train the entire bottom press. You can put your hands under your buttocks.

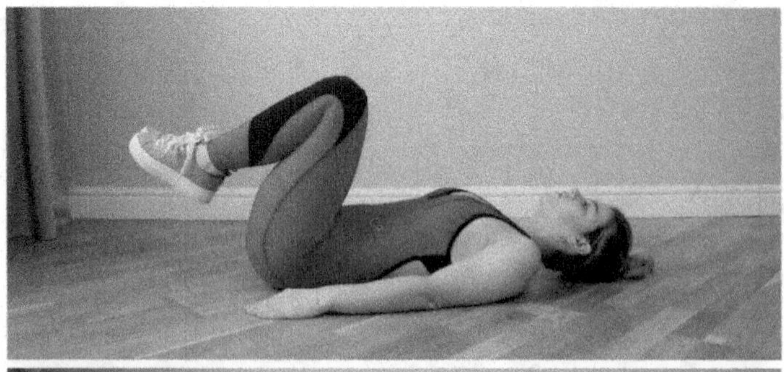

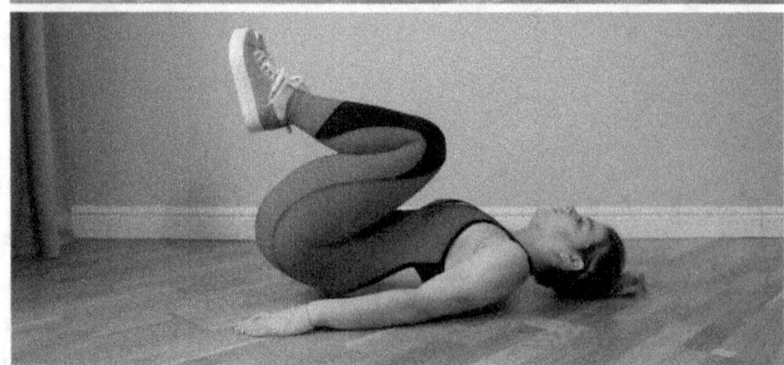

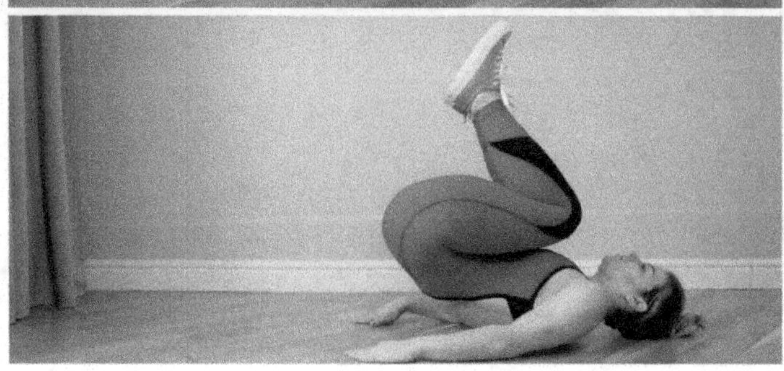

<u>12.10.</u> <u>Plank. Legs are led diagonally to the elbows.</u>

- The number of repetitions is 20 times.
- The essence of the exercise - the body is even; the arms are wider than the shoulders. Knees touch our hands in turn, as shown in the picture.

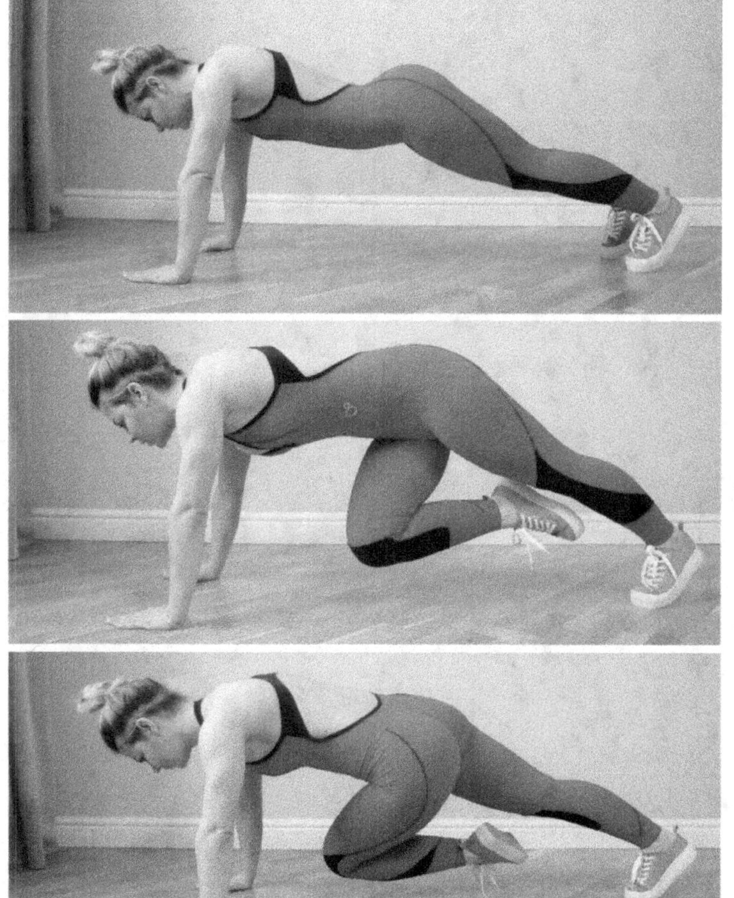

<u>12.11.</u>   <u>Plank. Lifting the legs 45 degrees alternately.</u>

- The number of repetitions is 20 times.
- The essence of the exercise - the body is even; the arms are wider than the shoulders. from this position, we raise our legs one by one, about 45 degrees. Perform the exercise as shown in the figure.in the picture.

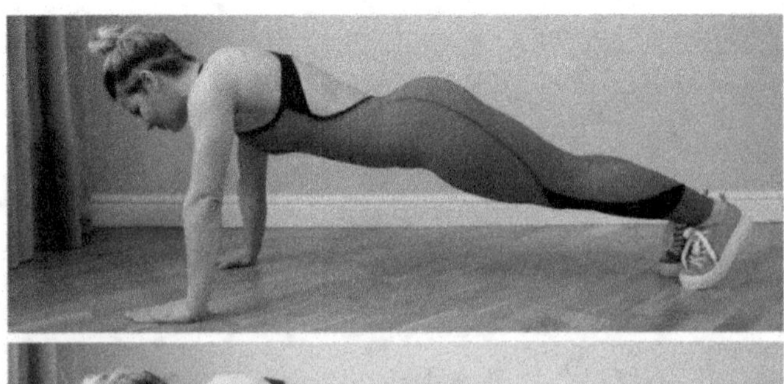

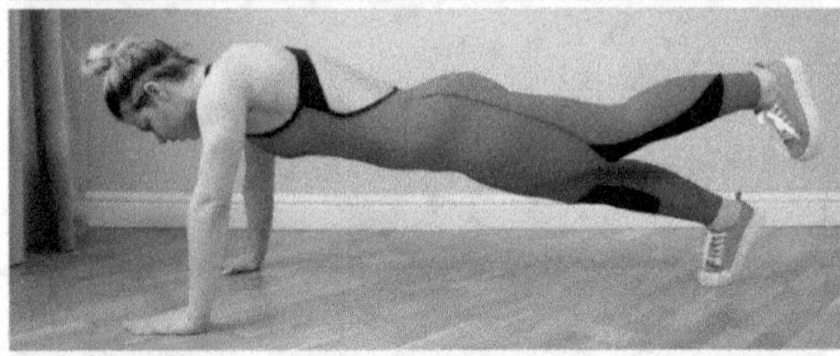

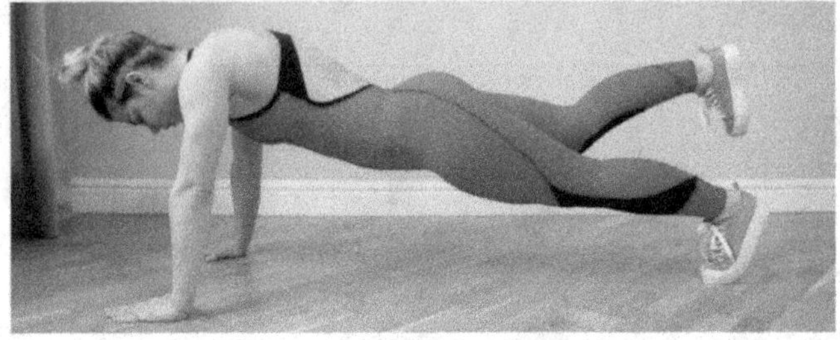

12.12. **<u>Plank. Moving his legs 45 degrees alternately to the sides.</u>**

- The number of repetitions is 20 times.
- The essence of the exercise - the body is even; The arms are wider than the shoulders. from this position, we alternately each foot performs a step to the side, about 45 degrees. Execute the exercise as shown in the figure.

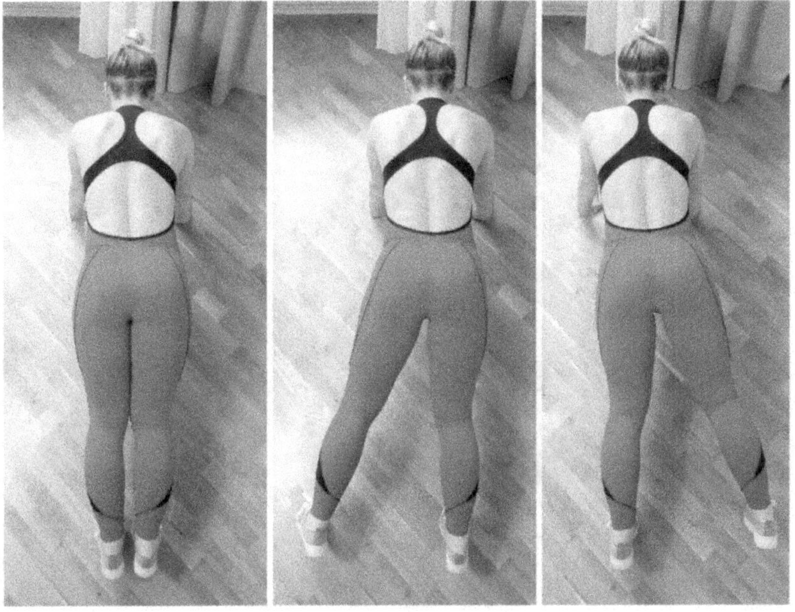

CHAPTER 13. Conclusion.

In conclusion of our sports booklet, firstly we want
to thank you for reading our book.
Secondly, we will be happy if you achieve great
results with our exercises and can share them with
us by writing us feedback or by sending a letter to
the mail julyyuliia@gmail.com .
You can write to us all your minds about exercises.

Our exercises for training upper body a were
useful to get this information.

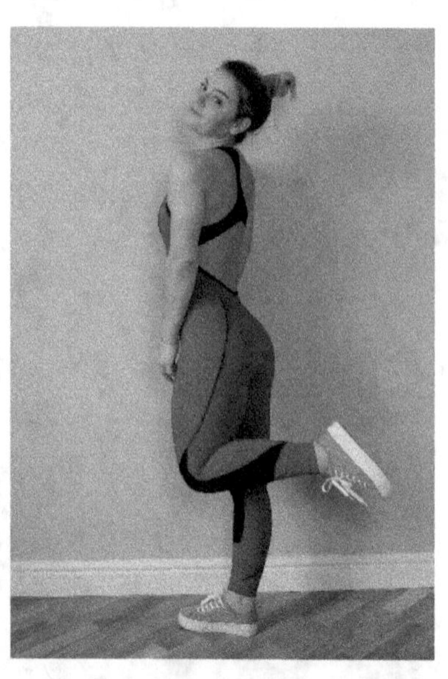

Julia is a supporter of bodybuilding, athlete,
fitness - coach of group programs, champion
in the category of "fitness bikini".

Thank you for reading.

www.ingramcontent.com/pod-product-compliance
Lightning Source LLC
Chambersburg PA
CBHW061519250726

48657CB00005B/1972